MW00984143

Published by Barbour Publishing, Inc., P.O. Box 719, Uhrichsville, Ohio 44683
www.barbourbooks.com

Member of the
Evangelical Christian
Publishers Association

Printed in China.

Get Well Soon!

GAIL SATTLER

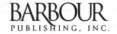

BARBOUR
PUBLISHING, INC.

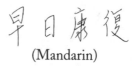

Get Well Soon!

Get Well Soon!
(English)

Com Os Desegos De Rapidas Melhoras!
(Portugese)

تمنى لك الشفاء سريع
(Lebanese)

Beste Wünsche Für Eine Baldige Genesung
(German)

早日康復
(Mandarin)

Get Well Soon!

Sièntase Mejor Pronto
(Spanish)

ਤੁਸੀ ਜਲਦੀ ਠੀਕ ਹੋ ਜਾਓ
(Punjabi)

J'espère Que Vous Sentir Mûr!
(French)

Скорого Виздоровлення
(Ukrainian)

Etgay Ellway Oonsay
(Pig Latin)

Friendship is a wonderful thing.
I value the time we spend together.
I value the time we spend apart,
Just knowing you're somewhere.
When you are not well, my heart aches.
I am thinking of you.

I am praying for you.

Praise the LORD, O my soul;
all my inmost being, praise his holy name.
Praise the LORD, O my soul,
and forget not all his benefits—
who forgives all your sins
and heals all your diseases,
who redeems your life from the pit
and crowns you with love and compassion,
who satisfies your desires with good things
so that your youth is renewed like the eagle's.

PSALM 103:1–5

1

God Made You!

Now is a good time to catch up on your reading.
—a quote from your church deacon

For you created my inmost being;
you knit me together in my mother's womb.
I praise you because
I am fearfully and wonderfully made;
your works are wonderful.
PSALM 139:13–14

. . .

*God made you.
Please take care of what
God has made.*

. . .

Wishing you flowers and sunshine,
Butterflies and birds that sing,
A return to good health,
And all the joy that will bring.

God created the heavens and the earth;
He created the plants, the animals
—every living thing.
God created splendor and beauty
Which man cannot comprehend,
And then, in all of His wondrous creation,
God made you, my friend.

. . .

*I'm sending you my prayers
and best wishes
for a speedy and complete recovery.*

Get Well Soon!

This is my Father's world,
O let me ne'er forget,
That tho' the wrong seems oft so strong,
God is the ruler yet.
This is my Father's world:
Why should my heart be sad?
The Lord is King—let the heavens ring;
God reigns; let the earth be glad
This is my Father's world!

"This Is My Father's World"
MALTBIE D. BABCOCK, 1901

2

Be Encouraged!

Chicken soup is good for what ails you.
—a quote from your concerned grandmother

Get Well Soon!

Instead of concentrating on being sick,
we can choose to think of what good can be accomplished
when we are forced to lie still.
I pray that you will experience peace in this time.
With peace comes healing, not just in our bodies,
but in our souls—where our thirst goes
beyond our physical needs.

. . .

Now if we are children, then we are heirs—heirs of
God and co-heirs with Christ,
if indeed we share in his sufferings
in order that we may also share in his glory.
ROMANS 8:17

Roses are red;
Violets are blue.
Because you need to get well,
I am praying for you.

. . .

*The LORD will sustain him
on his sickbed
and restore him from his bed of illness.*
PSALM 41:3

. . .

My hope is built on nothing less
Than Jesus' blood and righteousness. . . .
On Christ the solid Rock I Stand
"My Hope Is Built"
EDWARD MOTE, 1834

God is our refuge and strength,
an ever-present help in trouble.
Therefore we will not fear, though the earth give way
and the mountains fall into the
heart of the sea,
though its waters roar and foam
and the mountains quake with their surging.
PSALM 46:1–3

. . .

*God loves us too much to harm us,
and He's far too wise to make a mistake.*

. . .

When personal weakness begins to plague us,
that is a marvelous reminder.
God is our "very present help," our strength. Selah!
CHARLES R. SWINDOLL

And we know that in all things
God works for the good of those who love him,
who have been called according to his purpose.
For those God foreknew
he also predestined to be confirmed
to the likeness of his Son,
that he might be the firstborn among many brothers.
And those he predestined, he also called;
those he called, he also justified;
those he justified, he also glorified.
ROMANS 8:28–30

. . .

Never forget that God has called you unto Himself.
He has personally called you, inviting you to be His child.
God loves you that much.

Being fully persuaded that God truly loves you and
accepts you as you are, makes it easy to picture yourself
standing in His presence enjoying the pleasures that
are at His right hand that now belong to you.
ROY H. HICKES, D.D.

. . .

God loves you.
What more is there to say?

. . .

So do not fear, for I am with you;
do not be dismayed, for I am your God.
I will strengthen you and help you;
I will uphold you with my righteous right hand.
ISAIAH 41:10

3

Smile. It's good for you.

Smile awhile and give your face a rest.
—a quote sung by the man next door

A cheerful heart is good medicine.
PROVERBS 17:22

. . .

It is God's desire for us to have joyful hearts.
He wants us not only to be happy,
but to have joyful attitudes.
He wants us to live our lives to the fullest potential,
with Him in our hearts.
We all know that not every circumstance
is joyful or pleasant, but God is with us—
and with Him we can have a cheerful heart,
which is good medicine, indeed.

Get Well Soon!

I hope and pray that soon you will be
restored to your "old" self.
Not that you're old. That's just a saying.
Really. You can trust me. I'm your friend.
Methuselah lived 969 years (see Genesis 5:27).
That's old! Not you!

. . .

Being sick isn't all that bad.
First, you don't have to go to work.
No one bugs you to clean up your mess.
You don't have to answer the phone
unless you really want to.
The dog keeps your feet warm
when you can't find your slippers.

Smile, and the world smiles with you.
Cry, and you're going to need another box of tissues.

. . .

But the LORD made the heavens.
Splendor and majesty are before him;
strength and joy in his dwelling place.

1 CHRONICLES 16:26–27

. . .

A man asked his doctor if he would be able to play the
violin after his broken arm was healed and the cast
removed. The doctor assured him that he would,
and at the news, the man rejoiced. After all,
he'd never been able to play the violin before. . . .

4

Things To Do When You're Sick

Take two aspirin and call me in the morning.
—a quote from your family doctor

Get Well Soon!

Things to do when you're stuck in bed:

- See how the lumps of stucco on the bedroom ceiling can act as a sundial.
- Figure out exactly how many dogs are in your neighborhood by the barking.
- Count the number of tissues that are really in one box— just to make sure the manufacturer is honest.
- See how many days it takes for a glass of water to evaporate.
- Don't feel guilty about wearing socks in bed.

Humble yourselves, therefore, under God's mighty hand,
that he may lift you up in due time.
Cast all your anxiety on him because he cares for you.
1 PETER 5:6–7

. . .

Jesus can help no one who needs nothing.
RICHARD C. HALVERSON

. . .

Renew yourself as the days go by.
Each morning, hear the simple joy of the birds in the sky.
When comes the noon, the middle of the day,
The earth basks in the warmth of the sun's gentle rays.
When the day is over, the glowing sunset comes anew,
Each night praise God, for He has created you, too.

Get Well Soon!

Many of God's chosen people struggled with illnesses. Turn the page for the answers to these trivia questions.

1. Which prominent Bible figure prayed three times for a recurring physical condition to be removed?
2. Which great man of the Old Testament was hit with overwhelming depression?
3. Who said, "Lord, the one you love is sick"?
4. When Erastus stayed in Corinth and Paul went to Cos, who stayed behind in Miletus because he was sick?
5. Who had stomach problems, as well as other infirmities?

Get Well Soon!

Answers to quiz on page 25. . .

1. Paul had a chronic physical condition only named as "a thorn" in his flesh. (2 Corinthians 12:7–10)
2. Elijah slunk off into the desert in a deeply depressed state not long after a major victory. (1 Kings 19)
3. The sisters of Lazarus—Mary and Martha. (John 11:3)
4. Trophimus remained in Miletus due to illness. (2 Timothy 4:20)
5. Paul instructed Timothy to take wine for medicinal purposes. (1 Timothy 5:23)

Get Well Soon!

Things to think about when you're stuck in bed:

- Remember an old friendship.
- Think about calling or writing that person.
- And then do it.
- Reflect on a new friendship.
- Consider why that person is so special.
- And then call or write him, too.
- Think about someone who has hurt you.
- Think of why.
- Pray for her.

5

Thoughts

Turn that music off! You're supposed to be sick!
—a quote from your elderly neighbor

Get Well Soon!

Good things that can be accomplished when you're stuck in bed:

- You can lose weight.
- You gain loads of sympathy from friends and relatives.
- You see people you haven't seen for a long time when they bring you nice cards.
- You can catch up on all your reading.
- You can analyze the bedroom decor as never before.
- Memorize your favorite Scripture verse.
- Completely master all the remote controls.
- If you're crabby when you're sick, it will prove just how nice you really are on normal days.

The full flood of my life is not in bodily health,
not in external happenings,
not in seeing God's work succeed,
but in the perfect understanding of God,
and in the communion with Him that Jesus Himself had.
OSWALD CHAMBERS

. . .

*May each day bring you closer
to full health.*

Get Well Soon!

With the help of the thorn in my foot,
I spring higher than anyone with sound feet.
SØREN KIERKEGAARD

. . .

In bringing many sons to glory, it was fitting that God,
for whom and through whom everything exists,
should make the author of their salvation
perfect through suffering.
HEBREWS 2:10

. . .

A person who was suffering asked his pastor
why God had made him like that.
His reply,
"God has not made you; God *is making* you."

In other words, our Savior has gone through life,
has taken all of life's beatings and buffetings,
and He has gone before us. And now?
Now He pulls us toward Himself!
He invites His followers within the veil.
He says, "Come in. Find here the rest that you need,
the relief from the burdens and buffetings of doubt."

CHARLES R. SWINDOLL

. . .

As you journey along the path of recovery to good health,
Many good wishes are being sent your way,
That the journey is a quick one and you'll soon be
good as new.

Finally, brothers, whatever is true,
whatever is noble, whatever is right,
whatever is pure, whatever is lovely,
whatever is admirable—
if anything is excellent or praiseworthy—
think about such things.
PHILIPPIANS 4:8

. . .

*I look forward to the day
when you are well again.
I hope and pray it is soon.
Recover well, my friend.*

6

Wishes for You

When you're sick, I'm sad. I miss you. Get well soon.
—a quote from me, your friend

Get Well Soon!

Make God's Kingdom and His way of doing things
first in your life,
and He will give you everything you need.

FRITZ RIDENOUR

. . .

_May God's glory be shown
in the healing of your body,
mind, and spirit._

. . .

_He_ gives strength to the weary and
increases the power of the weak.

ISAIAH 40:29

But He said to me,
"My grace is sufficient for you, for my power is made
perfect in weakness." Therefore I will boast all the more
gladly about my weaknesses, so that Christ's power may
rest on me. That is why, for Christ's sake, I delight in
weaknesses, in insults, in hardships, in persecutions,
in difficulties. For when I am weak, then I am strong.

2 CORINTHIANS 12:9–10

. . .

May you be strong in your heart
as your body gains strength.
May you be energized as each day gets better
than the day before.
May you be encouraged with healing and recovery.
And may every day bless you more and more.

Life is a gift!

Life in itself is a gift from our almighty Father.
God has given us total freedom.
Along with the gift to experience and appreciate joy
and a sound body, we also are given the ability
to feel sickness and pain.
Without sadness, we would never know
the true meaning of joy.
Without sickness, we would never know
the true meaning of health.
I pray that you will use this time to pray and meditate,
and bring yourself into a deeper relationship
with our God, who is the Savior of us all.

Friends, family, and well-wishers have many ways
of expressing their best wishes to people
in times of illness.
Cards and flowers are the most common.
Others present books to those who are ill.
There are times when a book is too much,
but a card isn't enough.
I pray this gift book will be a special blessing to you,
a small way to show you
how special you are to me,
and how much I miss you when you are sick.
Get well soon, my friend.

My Prayer for You

My prayer for you is that you may seek the Lord in times of weakness and need. I pray you will find strength in His glory and His ultimate wisdom. I pray you will find continuing peace in His Word, and that you will never forget God's love for your. He sent His Son to take the punishment for all your sins.

May God give you strength and healing, and patience when you need it. Let this time not be a test but a time of renewal for you. I pray that good may be accomplished for you and in you, as nothing God allows to happen can be discounted.

May God bless you and keep you comforted, and most of all, I pray for God's healing touch upon you. Amen.

*I hope your path to recovery
is short and smooth,
with no bumps along the way.
My prayer for you is that you continue
to improve,
and that you are healed
a little more each day.*